I0424054

Beginner's Guide to
Exercise
and Better Health

Robert Berry

2

Table-Of-Contents

Introduction

Chapter 1 Reasons to Exercise

Chapter 2 Procrastination and Motivation

Chapter 3 Exercising at Home

Chapter 4 Exercising at the Gym

Chapter 5 Maintaining the Momentum

Conclusion

Exercise Glossary

This document is geared towards providing exact and reliable information in regards to the topic and issue covered. The publication is sold with the idea that the publisher is not required to render accounting, officially permitted, or otherwise, qualified services. If advice is necessary, legal or professional, a practiced individual in the profession should be ordered.

- From a Declaration of Principles which was accepted and approved equally by a Committee of the American Bar Association and a Committee of Publishers and Associations.

In no way is it legal to reproduce, duplicate, or transmit any part of this document in either electronic means or in printed format. Recording of this publication is strictly prohibited and any storage of this document is not allowed

Introduction

Exercise.

It's a scary word for many of us.

For some, it conjures up unpleasant memories of under achieving embarrassment during those excruciating PE sessions that we've spent years trying to erase from our minds.

It is associated with pain, fatigue, exhaustion and all kinds of other unpleasantness.

And it has always been something we sucked at.

Imagine though if exercise was different. Imagine if it was something that you looked forward to. Imagine if it was your special time to maintain, shape and create the type of body and mind that you know you deserve to live inside of. Imagine if exercise was the vehicle to a new, enhanced, more vibrant, self fulfilled version of yourself.

You don't have to imagine because exercise is precisely that. It always has been. The problem has been that too few people have had the key to unlocking the door to exercise fulfillment. This book will provide you with that key.

There's a massive industry that has been created over the exercise 'craze' of the past 40 years. It has made billions of dollars for a lot of fat investors and, along the way perpetuated a whole litany of lies about what it takes to get fit and lose weight. Foremost among them is the belief that you need to join a gym to get in shape.

In the pages to follow, we'll dispel many of the common misconceptions about exercise, weight loss and getting in shape. In the process, we will provide you with everything you need to get started and progressing to a forever-fit future.

Chapter 1: Reasons to Exercise

We've always known that working out was a smart thing to do, but recently there have been a whole host of studies that back up just how beneficial getting some sweat in your day can be for you. There is nothing else that you could do, no pill, food or supplement that you can take that will offer you results comparable to regular exercise.

For a lot of people it's easy to find reasons why you can't exercise. It's now time to flip that coin and start thinking about reasons why you can – and should – commit to regular exercise. In this chapter we will list 50 reasons why you need to get into the exercise habit. Use this list as a motivational resource for when you're feeling uninspired and just can't seem to pull yourself off that couch.

Exercise will do the following for you:

> ➢ Improve your Mood

> ➢ Make it easier for you to learn

- ➢ Build self-esteem
- ➢ Keep you grain fit
- ➢ Keep you fit, functional and agile
- ➢ Improve your mental well being
- ➢ Heighten your immune system
- ➢ Reduce your stress level
- ➢ Bring happiness
- ➢ Slows down the aging process
- ➢ Gives you a better quality of sleep
- ➢ Enhance joint mobility
- ➢ Gives you better skin tone and color
- ➢ Ward off strokes
- ➢ Makes you stronger
- ➢ Reduces anxiety
- ➢ Improves your memory
- ➢ Help you kick unhealthy addictions
- ➢ Makes you more productive

- ➢ Improves your creative thinking ability
- ➢ Improve your body image
- ➢ Boost confidence
- ➢ Helps keep you focused
- ➢ Improve your nutritional practices
- ➢ Make your bones stronger
- ➢ Make your heart stronger
- ➢ Increases longevity
- ➢ Give you better posture
- ➢ Prevents colds and flu
- ➢ Improves appetite
- ➢ Reduce bad cholesterol levels
- ➢ Lowers the risk of certain cancers
- ➢ Bring down high blood pressure
- ➢ Fight depression
- ➢ Reduce diabetes risk
- ➢ Fights dementia
- ➢ Reduces back pain
- ➢ Decreases the risk of osteoporosis

- ➢ Protect muscle tissue
- ➢ Boost energy levels
- ➢ Enhance sporting ability
- ➢ Boost pain tolerance
- ➢ Enhance balance and stability
- ➢ Enhance oxygen uptake
- ➢ Boost concentration levels
- ➢ Helps you to be more self controlled
- ➢ Reduce fatigue levels
- ➢ Enhance libido
- ➢ Allows you to shape your body your way
- ➢ Improve the overall quality of your life

Having considered this exhaustive list of benefits, you now know just how valuable regular exercise time really is. Yet, despite the many intrinsic rewards that come with exercising, the vast majority of people work out because they want to look better. And the majority of them want to exercise to help them to lose weight. So, let's take a moment to find out just how exercise can help you on your journey to a new, slimmer you.

Your body is constantly managing the balance between energy intake and energy expenditure. You take energy in in the form of food and you expend it by way of your basal metabolic rate and physical activity. The difference between the two is your net energy balance. If intake exceeds expenditure, then a positive net energy balance occurs and energy gets stored as body fat.

The energy expenditure of your body depends upon . . .
- ✓ Your starting body weight
- ✓ Your basal metabolic rate
- ✓ Physical activity

The level of physical activity is dependent upon the following factors:

- ➢ Frequency of the activity

- ➢ The intensity of the exercise

- ➢ The duration of the activity

➤ The type of activity performed

By creating a negative net energy balance through exercise, you will lose body fat. Of course, this pre-supposes that you don't eat extra calories to offset the amount of calories burned through the exercise that you are doing. For example, it would take a person 30 minutes of moderate walking to burn off the calories in a plain donut.

Coupled with a proper nutritional program, the right type of exercise will allow you to lose body fat consistently as you strip away the layers to reveal a leaner, meaner you.

The basic recommendations for physical activity are 150 minutes per week of moderate intensity exercise. That equates to about half an hour a day, five days a week. Recent studies, however, indicate that more is better. Our bodies were not designed to sit around all day under artificial light tapping away at a keyboard.

We were made to move, to jump and to run. No magic pill, vitamin, drug or app can negate that simple fact.

By embracing a lifestyle which is grounded in fitness and exercise, you will be giving yourself the greatest gift of all – a fuller, more satisfying life.

Chapter 2: Procrastination and Motivation

It's the eternal dilemma.

Instant gratification versus long-term benefit:

Mouth watering muffin versus a lowered cholesterol level in old age.

Cookies and Cream Ice-cream versus fitting into your jeans.

Triple sundae with chocolate sauce versus lowering your risk of Type 2 Diabetes.

Let's be honest about it – instant gratification has a lot going for it, particularly when we are living in a world that is unfailingly giving the message to indulge our every whim. Unless we're able to identify the real reasons behind our weight loss efforts, we'll never rise above the instant-noodles society that has spawned the obesity epidemic that threatens the Western World. So, let's start digging . . .

So you want to exercise?

Great.

But before we go any further it's imperative that you discover why you want to exercise.

To lose weight?

Why do you want to lose weight?

When you discover what drives you, you'll also know what motivates you. If you don't identify your inner driver, it doesn't matter how hard you try, how much sweat you expend or how many calories you burn, you will fail. Uncovering the reason that you really want to achieve your goal attaches an emotional element to that goal. And the more emotional content you can stir up, the more motivated you'll be to go after it. Remember the words of German philosopher Friedrich Nietzsche . . .

He who has a why to live can bear almost any how.

Getting emotionally involved with your goal will deeply impress your why into your subconscious. The subconscious is the seat of your unthinking actions - your habits. Every message that filters through to it is accepted without question and acted upon automatically. That is exactly where you want your weight maintenance habits to be because the subconscious always expresses itself in physical form - positive behaviors that will reinforce your goal.

The reasons for exercising are many. As we've seen in the last chapter. Your goal may not to be lose weight. In the remainder of this sectiion, however, we are going to assume that weight loss is the goal. It could in fact be the opposite – to gain muscular body weight.

Stop and ask yourself right now, just why you want to lose weight. Here are a couple of key questions to help you identify that reason:

> 1. What is important to you about reaching your weight goal?

> 2. How will your life be better after you have achieved your weight goal?

For some people, looking their absolute best for an upcoming event, such as a wedding, is their emotional motivator. For others it is to be able to be an active, healthy role model for their kids. Others may find that their emotional drive comes from maintaining their sex appeal in the eyes of their partner. Once you have found your emotional driver, write it down in the following format . . .

The emotional driver behind my weight loss goal is to . . . . When I have achieved my goal I will feel . . .

Once you have identified the emotional driver to your goal, it is time to reinforce it by adding in a spiritual element. It doesn't matter whether you are a believer in a Creator, an atheist or an agnostic. Spirituality involves being in touch with your reason for being. Whether you were created, evolved or were placed here by aliens, you have ended up with a magical, unique and highly intricate machine that will govern your state of well-being until you die. Those who do believe in a Creator God have an obligation to Him to respect and maintain the amazing body that they have been gifted. All of us owe it to ourselves to identify the spiritual reason that accompanies our goal. Find out what yours is and keep yourself accountable to it.

Now that you've discovered the emotional and spiritual drivers that will motivate you toward your goal, it's time to learn how to apply the goal setting formula that will catapult you toward your end game.

Five Steps to Goal Achievement

1. Set Specific Goals - Losing weight is not a goal. It's far too general. Body weight is composed of muscle, water, minerals, vitamins and fat, among other things. Your only ambition is to lose body fat. But even that goal has to be narrowed down. If you focus on the specific behaviors that will bring about your desired fat loss and set them as your goals, then the fat loss will take care of itself. Your goals, then, should be to do with the actions and habits that

will keep you on your weight management plan.

2. Set Measurable Goals - Unless you have a means of measuring your progress regularly you will struggle to maintain your motivation. Don't expect yourself to make the transition from cookie munching couch potato to fitness / nutrition junkie in a couple of weeks. Set behavior related goals that build upon each other and widen out to encompass all aspects of a healthy lifestyle.

3. Set Stepping Stone Goals - You definitely need a long-term goal - your ultimate physical look. But it's also imperative that you break that goal down, working backwards to yearly, 3 monthly, weekly and daily goals. Your 3 monthly goal should revolve around such behaviors as recording your food intake and exercise every day, or increasing your cardio exercise duration by 15 minutes per day by walking at a slightly uncomfortable pace. Your daily and weekly goals should

revolve around the exercise and eating disciplines that are immediately before you.

4. Record Your 3 Month Goal - Write your 3 month goal on a business sized card and get it laminated. Write your goal in the present tense as if it has already taken place. Here's the wording . . .

   *The date is (date in 3 months time), and I am now doing every*thing *I can to get me to my desired weight, including recording my daily food intake and workouts every day.*

   Now that you have your card you need to carry it with your everywhere your go. Every 90 minutes make sure that you pull it out and read it to yourself.

5. Visualize Your Goals - One of the most interesting innovations in sports psychology over recent times has been the rise of visualization, or mental rehearsal. Sports teams the world-over are

using it to build an unconquerable mental drive toward goal attainment. But you don't need to go out and hire a sports psychologist to benefit from the power of visulaization. You can do it on your own by mentally rehearsing the achievment of your goals. Start at the daily level and do it while you are lying in bed. See yourself doing everything that you need to in order to have a perfect goal attainment day, from springing out of bed, enjoying a healthy nutritious breakfast, powering through an invigorating, calorie depleting work-out and then enjoying an energy restoring post work-out shake.

Now that you have your emotional, spiritual and mental underpinning for your goals and have learnt exactly how to go about setting proper goals, it's time to make a record of your goals:

1) Create a Goal Setting document and record your goals on a time-line, starting with your daily goal and

ending with your ultimate body goal.
2) Type up, print out and laminate your 3 monthly goals.

You now have a roadmap to turning every endeavour, every goal, every quest into an unquestionable reality. You are able to unleash the power of your subconscious in conjunction with your mind muscle connection to become unstoppable. So, get out there and claim what's yours!

How to Defeat Procrastination

Procrastination affects all of us. We seem to have an inbuilt tendency to put off the things we know we have to do, even when we appreciate how good they are for us. Here are 3 powerful techniques to prevent procrastination sabotaging your exercise ambitions:

> **The Ten Minute Rule** – If we perceive that a job is going to be hard work, we develop an aversion to it in our minds that leads us to keep putting it off. However, when we break the larger task down into

smaller, more manageable chunks, it suddenly becomes much easier to think about. With your exercise sessions, rather than thinking of a 34 minute workout, chunk it out to a 7 minute warm up, 10 minutes of resistance training, 10 minutes of cardio and then a 7 minute warm down. This makes the task seem far easier to achieve.

> **Three Magical Questions** – Next time you procrastinate in the face of an important assignment, take a piece of paper and answer 3 simple questions . . .

1) Where are you?

2) What do you want to do?

3) How will you feel after doing the task?

The very act of putting the task down in writing will make you visualize yourself already doing it. Then it's simply a matter of your body following through with the task.

> **Ultimate Goal VS Immediate Desire** – The battle between long

term goal and immediate desire is always going to be a losing proposition for the goal. But, you can win in this standoff every time by simply making your ultimate goal and you immediate desire switch places. Turn your immediate desire into something you can put off until later. Then make your ultimate goal into something that you insist on right now. Ask yourself this question . . .

At this moment would I prefer good health or junk food?

Learning to Love Exercise

Forget the Past

Over 70% of Americans are either sedentary or not receiving the minimum amount of recommended exercise. Despite knowing that they should be working out, a lot of these people simply don't like exercise. This attitude is typically formed very early on in life.

By putting aside the bad experiences you have had in the past and focusing on new things that you find enjoyable, you'll be able to make your mind over. The key is to find an activity that you really enjoy doing and use it as the foundation for your exercise session.

Pace Yourself

When you first start working out, don't go full out straight away. If you exhaust yourself straight off the bat, you'll be adding fuel to the idea that you don't like exercising. Take it steady and build up gradually, enjoying the training along the way.

Exercise is movement. It's not confined to the gym or a set block of workout time. It could be walking, swimming, playing basketball or any other activity that you enjoy that will get your heart rate up for 30 minutes.

Ditch the Excuses

A lot of people tell themselves that they don't have time for exercise. We're all incredibly busy with more and more demands coming in on us all the time. But, exercise needs to be a priority in your schedule. It is, after all, the key to everything else. Unless your body is maintained you will not be able to do all of those other things that are tugging at your time. For that reason you must schedule your workout into your calendar as non-negotiable 'you' time. Let people know that you are not available during those times.

Sometimes we have excellent intentions to exercise, but simply can't build up the motivation. The key, again, is to find something that you enjoy doing. If you enjoy it, motivation will not be a problem. A great way to overcome lack of motivation is to ask a friend to be your workout buddy. If you know that someone is waiting for you, you're much more likely to turn up at the exercise venue than if you're just relying on your own motivation level to get you there.

A trap that people often fall into is to put barriers in front of their ability to exercise. They do this by telling themselves that they must buy something before they can begin. It could be new shoes, gym clothes or a stopwatch that they have told themselves they need before they can start training. These are really just ways to procrastinate.

The reality is that you don't need any special equipment in order to get started on an exercise routine. Put the excuses aside, save your money, and just get started.

Overcome Insecurities

A lot of people feel very self-conscious when it comes to exercise. They can easily let their own personal insecurities hold them back. They'll convince themselves that others will laugh at them. That is almost certainly not going to be the case. If you've felt these insecurities, you simply have to put aside what you think other people might be thinking and just go ahead and do the things that you've always wanted to do.

Variety is the Spice of Fitness

The key to overcoming boredom while exercising is variety. Mixing up your exercise will keep you feeling fresh and engaged. If you've been lifting weights your whole life, try out yoga or pilates. The more you mix it and add variety to your training, the less likely it is that you'll get bored or injured or plateau.

Variety is also the key to progress within your workout. Your body is an amazing machine that is able to quickly adapt to the type of stresses that you place upon it. When it comes to exercise, however, adaptation is not what you want. You want to keep your body guessing, to keep making it work in new and different ways. Then it will be forced to work differently in order to improve.

As a result of the need to add variety to your exercise routine, you should not continue on a workout program for more than six weeks. Changing it up will keep your body and your mind stimulated.

Chapter 3: Exercising at Home

(In this chapter and the one to follow, we'll be presenting a range of workouts. You will find complete exercise descriptions in the glossary at the end of this e-book).

You don't have to join a gym to get fit. Despite what many people think and what the multi billion-dollar fitness industry promotes, exercise isn't about the right pair of shoes, the right app or the right training studio. It's about two things only, and they are both absolutely free of charge . . .

Your Body.

Gravity.

Your Body

Your body contains all of the equipment you'll ever need to get lean, muscular and aerobically in top condition. Granted your body-weight will not turn you into Mr. Olympia, but it will allow you to develop a physique that will turn heads. Don't believe me – take a look at a top competitive gymnast. I bet you'll see a body that you'd kill for. Well, it was developed with just two things – the gymnast's own body weight and the second crucial element in the fit success equation– gravity.

With nothing more than your birthday suit and the power of gravity, I'm going show you how to achieve awesome workouts that get results. We are going to focus on the two key fitness systems of your body to ensure complete, overall health, well-being and peak development. Those two systems are the aerobic and the anaerobic systems.

Gravity

Gravity is a wonderful thing. As well as keeping stuff anchored to the surface of the earth, it allows you to get a great workout with nothing but your own body weight. With nothing but what you were born with you are able to build muscle mass and strength, increase muscular endurance and lose fat.

There are some obvious benefits of body weight training as opposed to making use of either free weights or machines.

1) You don't have to spend a small fortune to get your workout in

2) You can work out anywhere, any time

3) The movement is natural and functional – you aren't restricted or placed in a fixed position

4) The movements are functional, allowing you to emulate the real movements that you perform throughout the day

Your Home Gym Bodyweight Workouts

In this section, we will discuss the components that make up an effective bodyweight program. We'll also provide some guidelines on how you can maximize the potential of your body as your gym, along with some vital safety precautions that will prevent your 'equipment' from breaking down on you.

Push / Pull Training

There are two basic ways to train your body. You either pull towards your body or you push away from your body. Due to the force of gravity, body weight training has traditionally been heavily weighted towards Push training. Push movements like push ups are more convenient than Pull movements like pull ups. All you need to do is lower yourself to the ground and then push back to the starting position.

Unless you balance your training between Pushing and Pulling, however, you will fail to achieve the balanced development and functional strength that you need for overall strength, muscularity and fitness. That is why bodyweight pulling movements are an important part of this program. This will require the use of some form of pull up bar which you can grip in order to pull your body away from the ground. You can use a beam in your garage, a home chin up bar door attachment or you can make your own chin up apparatus.

Modified pull up movements are a stepping-stone to full pull ups. These can be performed with a bar (broomstick handle?) and a couple of chairs.

Most bodyweight training programs that you'll find neglect the training of the muscles of the back. That is a mistake. Without strong latissimus, rhombus and erector spinae muscles, you will open yourself up to structural imbalance problems, along with rounded shoulders, anterior pelvic tilt and lower back pain. In this program we will creatively utilize variations of pulling exercises to ensure balanced development of the muscles of both the front and back of your body.

Train Hard, Train Safe

An effective bodyweight training program requires that you make use of everyday furniture that you have around your home. This may include a door frame, a chair or table top. It is vital that every piece of training equipment that you use is secure, stable and strong. Always stabilize items before using them. Do a couple of test repetitions before doing your actual set in order to test rigidity.

Bodyweight training is a very safe way to work out when compared to what goes on in most gyms. Still, one unwise move can plunge you into a world of pain – and frustration. Follow these guidelines to ensure that you are training safe while training hard:

Don't Over Train

Your muscles don't grow when you train. Unless you provide sufficient time for the muscle to recover before working it again, you will never make progress. Not providing your connective tissues time to recover between workouts can set you up for problems. For those reasons, you should give your body 48 hours recovery between doing the same exercise again.

Use Perfect Form

In this book, you will learn the optimum form to allow you to maximize your training effort on every exercise. You must have the focus and discipline to use this proper form on every repetition. Don't just focus on reaching a total number of reps. Make sure that your body is moving through a full range of motion, especially on movements like push ups. Poor form is the number one cause of injury.

Balance Your Training

Your body is designed to work as a whole unit. If you train certain parts and not others, you will develop imbalances which will inevitably translate to injury. Your best protection against chronic injury, then, is balanced, strength, balanced flexibility and balanced muscle mass.

Stop When It Feels Wrong

There's a fine line between being focused on hitting your rep target and using common sense when you feel pain. There is no sense in pushing through unnatural pain (as opposed to muscular fatigue) to finish your set. If you don't give your body the respect it deserves, you may find yourself unable to train for weeks, defeating the purpose of what you're doing. So, listen to your body.

Warm Up

The erroneous idea that bodyweight training is not serious training can lead people to skip the warm up. This is a mistake. You need to warm up to move your body from cold, and rigid to warm and flexible. The colder a muscle is, the more prone it is to injury. Spend a few minutes gradually getting your heart rate up with jogging on the spot, jumping jacks or skipping. Warm up the particular muscles that you will be working by doing static stretches for them.

Focus

Too many people exercise mindlessly. They may be thinking about what happened at work that day, what they've still got to accomplish before bed or what's for dinner, but not about what they are actually doing. Yet, unless you are tuned in to the movement that you are currently performing you will not get the most out of it. You will also be increasing your risk of injury. That's why it is crucial that you develop what is known as the mind-muscle connection. Focus on the prime mover of the exercise. For example, when performing push ups, focus on the feeling across your pectoral muscles. Feel them stretching, expanding and contracting. Imagine them as pistons, mechanically driving up and down.

Slow Down

Most people exercise too fast. They have a 'get it over with' mentality that leads to partial movements and sloppy form. Just watch people doing push ups and you'll see what I mean. They pump out quarter movements, dropping their head to limit the range of motion, at about 3 per second. They may as well have not bothered. To get the most out of your exercise, perform the concentric (positive part) of the movement to a 2-second count. The eccentric (negative) part should take 3 seconds.

Sample Bodyweight Home Training Program

Complete this program as a circuit, doing 12 repetitions on each exercise. Do not rest between exercises. At the end of the circuit rest for exactly two minutes and then do it again. Work up to completing 4 circuits of the program:

Push Ups

Skipping x 30 seconds

Modified Pull Ups

Skipping x 30 seconds

Reverse Dips

Skipping x 30 seconds

Bodyweight Squats

Box Jumps

Skipping x 30 seconds

Mason Crunches

Skipping x 30 seconds

Jumping Split Lunges

Setting Up a Home Gym

There are some obvious advantages to having your own home gym:

- ✓ You don't have to commute to the gym
- ✓ You don't have to hunt for a park
- ✓ You don't have to wait around for equipment
- ✓ You don't have to contend with unsanitary conditions
- ✓ You don't have to make a recurring monthly payment
- ✓ You are not locked into a nightmarish contract

Despite the advantages of the home options, many people shy away from the idea, thinking that it will be cost prohibitive. However, the home fitness market has really 'grown up' in the last decade, and there is now a range of equipment available that is high quality and cost effective. It is now possible to put together a comprehensive home training facility that will give you a gym equivalent workout.

Some people have the luxury of a dedicated space for their home gym. It may be a basement, a portion of the garage or an attic. For others, the gym has to be of a stow-away kind, that can be quickly dismantled and slid away, out of sight. Let's consider both options.

The Portable Home Gym

Not so long ago, portable home fitness equipment was junk. It was cheap, mass produced, gimmicky and unreliable. While you can still find plenty of that type of equipment, you can also find gear that is manufactured to the highest standard using premium grade materials. And, even better, they are not cost prohibitive. These pieces of equipment are portable and easy to set up and take down. In fact, it is now possible to transform any space, including your living room, into your own workout studio in just a few minutes.

Here's how . . .

Essential Equipment:

- ✓ TRX Suspension training system
- ✓ Doorway Pull Up Bar

✓ Resistance Bands

✓ Adjustable dumbbells

✓ Stability Ball

✓ Skipping rope

✓ Exercise mat

TRX Suspension Training System

Suspension training has revolutionized the personal fitness space. It allows you to do a whole lot of things with your body and gravity that you can't do alone. In fact, a suspension trainer will allow you to perform in excess of 300 exercises that will hit every muscle group in your body.

A suspension trainer is made up of a combination of straps, cords and buckles that attaches to a closed doorway to provide you with a push / pull resistance that replaces dozens of bulky gym machines. By manipulating the leverage of the straps, you are able to provide yourself with a range of resistance levels to suit your every need. To make the movement harder, you simply shorten the length of the strap.

Suspension Trainers have been around since 2005, when former Navy Seal Randy Hetrick introduced his TRX system. The TRX has gone on to become the best selling and best regarded suspension training system on the market.

You'll pay around $200 for a good suspension training system. It's an investment that you won't regret.

Doorway Pull Up Bar

Often referred to as the upper body squat, the pull up is the single best exercise that you can perform to build a strong, muscular upper body. No gym is complete without a sturdy, reliable platform from which to perform pull ups. Fortunately, the market features a number of brands, which offer premium quality at an affordable price.

Doorway pull up bars come as either a telescopic single bar model or a door way mounted model. Telescopic bars have a winding portion which is unwound to secure the bar between the door opening. The doorway mounted version features a mounting bracket which sits on the door frame molding at the top reverse of the door. The doorway pull up bar offers more options and is generally sturdier than the telescopic bar and is the version that is recommended for your portable home gym.

A quality door way pull up bar can be yours for around $50.

Resistance Bands

Resistance bands have been around forever. For a long time, though, they were in the gimmicky exercise category. In the last few years, though, resistance bands have also grown up. Resistance bands offer some unique benefits over any other type of resistance training:

> ➤ They are lightweight, flexible and portable
> ➤ They are a great travel workout solution
> ➤ They allow for a freer range of motion than gravity bound equipment, allowing you to work from unique angles.

➢ They train muscles through both the positive and the negative range of an exercise.

Resistance tube bands come in various thicknesses and are usually color coded in accordance with the relative resistance level of the band. Many bands come with easy grip handles. The bands provide a restoring force, which is similar to a spring loaded weight machine. However, with bands, the force only comes into play when the ends of the band are pulled apart. So, the greater the extension of the band the greater the resistance. This type of training is known as linear resistance exercise. It has been scientifically shown provide a more targeted workout to fast twitch muscle fibers, which are primarily responsible for the development of muscular power.

Resistance bands generally follow a standard color-coded resistance level as follows:

➢ Level 1 (yellow) = 10 lbs.
➢ Level 2 (green) = 20 lbs.
➢ Level 3 (red) = 25 lbs.
➢ Level 4 (blue) = 30 lbs.

- ➢ Level 5 (extra heavy) = 35 lbs.
- ➢ Level 6 (extra, extra heavy) = 40 lbs.

Adjustable Dumbbells

One of the challenges of working out at home has to do with adding resistance, as you get stronger. Progressive resistance is at the heart of exercise success. That means that, as you get stronger, you need to add weight in order to keep making progress. In the gym, that's easy –just grab the next heaviest weight. But, when you're training at home it's a whole different story. To keep making progress, you have got to go and buy more weight. That becomes an expensive hassle.

Adjustable dumbbells are the smart solution to this problem. They allow you to change the resistance of the weight with a simple click of a dial. Adjustable dumbbells are actually just one set of dumbbells that sit on a special bed that allows you to select the resistance, which usually provides options from 5 through to about 80 pounds.

As well as providing an economical easy to be able to train with a range of different dumbbell weights, adjustable dumbbells allow you to have a complete weight set without having to take up a whole wall of space. That makes then compact, as well as affordable.

You can pick up a set of adjustable dumbbells for around $300. It may seem like a lot, and will probably be the biggest investment of you portable gym, but it will provide you with a dumbbell capability that would otherwise cost more than $2000.00.

Fitness Ball

A fitness ball, otherwise known as a Swiss ball, will allow you to do a lot of core exercises that will strengthen your lower back as your abs and intercostals shape up. It's also a great tool for increasing your flexibility. In addition, you can use the ball as your exercise bench when doing pressing movements with dumbbells. Doing so will allow you to work all of the small stabilizer muscles that are normally not activated when you do work on a flat bench.

Here's why you need to add a fitness ball to your portable training arsenal . . .

> ➤ The flexible, tactile surface allows you to get into advantageous positions that you can't achieve without it. These positions trick the body into working productively against its own weight or an external resistance. When you do the dumbbell chest press on the fitness ball, for example, you are not only working your chest, deltoids and triceps, but you are using every major muscle to hold your body in position on the ball.

> ➤ Due to the unstable nature of the ball, the body generates involuntary muscle actions / activity which allows you to target muscles that would ordinarily be less involved if the same movement was performed on a solid platform.

> ➤ Why is a fitness ball a great way to work the muscles of the core? The lumbopelvic region consists of the deep torso muscles,

transversus abdominus, multifidus, internal obliques and the layers of muscle and fascia that make up the pelvic floor. They are key to the active support of the lumbar spine, but, unfortunately they are also the most vulnerable to injury if neglected. Using a fitness ball as a semi-stable platform to support the body when doing strength and conditioning exercises recruits these muscles and is particularly productive because the muscle activity is involuntary so, rather than having to tell the body to do something, it simply gets on with the work that is required. In fact, these muscles are recruited a split second before any movements of the limbs, which suggests that the muscle actually anticipates the force that will soon be going through the lumbar spine.

Skipping

If you thought that skipping was just for little girls, then you're in for a major surprise . . . it turns out that jumping rope – skipping – is the most effective physical activity that you can engage in to lose fat, improve your cardiovascular fitness and get in the shape of your life.

So, what's so good about skipping? First and foremost, it melts fat away. The calories burned through every minute of jumping rope are on par with a strenuous game of basketball or a six-minute mile run.

At 14 calories churned through per minute, skipping is a mega fat burner. But not only that, skipping has been shown to induce the EPOC effect. EPOC stands for excess post exercise energy consumption. It means that you actually burn more calories after your skipping session has finished. So, skip for 20 minutes, and your metabolism rocks into overdrive, transforming your system into a fat burning furnace for the next 24-hours.

Another great plus for skipping is that it is so portable and convenient. Grab your rope and find a four square foot space and you're good to go – anywhere any time. This convenience factor is crucial to the one thing that will make or break your body transformations plans – regularity. With skipping, there are simply no excuses – and, believe me, that's a good thing!

Skipping is a low impact plyometric activity. This makes it a safe alternative for those who have suffered Achilles tendon issues from running or knee complaints from cycling. With skipping, you can get in a killer workout with minimum stress on the body.

Skipping is amazingly time efficient. After all, which would you rather do – run 8 miles in an hour or skip for 10 minutes? Skipping will reap the same benefits, while handing you back 50 minutes to spend on whatever you wish.

Maybe you're into weight training to build your body. Skipping will alow you to strip away bodyfat and bring out the definition in your muscles. If you want to really get ripped, showing off your newly built muscle to maximum effect, skip for 30 seconds between sets. You will lean out faster than you ever though possible.

Skipping will get you in the shape – and look – of your life. But, make no mistake – we're not advocating double-dutch here. Fitness skipping will push you to your limits, calling on all of your reserves of energy, determination and endurance. And don't worry if you've convinced yourself that you can't skip. Skipping is not something that you're born with – it's a learned activity. After a week, you'll be well and truly on your way. You don't have to learn to do fancy tricks, either. The basic two-footed jump with a single rope pass at moderate speed is a fantastic exercise. If you never learn any other way to skip, this one move will get you in better shape than 90% of the population.

You can pick up a very good skipping rope for $15.00

Exercise Mat

You'll need a quality exercise mat for your portable workout space. It will save your living environment from sweat while giving you a more comfortable surface on which to sweat. Make sure that the mat that you select features a sturdy grip on the underside that will not slip when you're using it. On the top side, you need a surface that won't sling to your body. Ideal mat thickness is about 1.8 inches. The best mats for in home use are made from thermal plastic elastomer.

A quality exercise mat will cost you around $20.00.

Making the Most of Your Portable Gym

Having gathered together the seven parts of your portable home gym, you are now ready to train your way to a new, improved you. Each piece of equipment described above is easily transportable, sets up in seconds and can be quickly stored away when the session is over. The following tips will allow you to get the most out of your portable gym.

- ✓ Set a schedule for your training. Try to have your sessions at the same time each day.

- ✓ Exercise when there are as few distractions in your life as possible. Early in the morning is good for many people.

- ✓ If training first thing in the morning, set up your portable gym the evening before. Install the doorway pull up bar and suspension system. Lay out your exercise map and position the adjustable dumbbell, resistance bands and fitness ball ready to go. Place a sweat towel by your mat and pop a water bottle in the fridge. In the morning, you'll be able to get straight into your session.

✓ Exercise on alternate days, giving your body plenty of time to rest and recuperate.

✓ Buy a monthly or yearly planner and display it on your wall. Mark off each workout as you complete it. The visual reinforcement of seeing your goal systematically being attained is a great form of daily motivation.

Sample Portable Gym Fitness Program (3 x per week on alternate days)

> *Warm Up – 5 minutes skipping*
> *Suspension Push Ups – 3 x 10-15 repetitions*

- *Pull Ups – 3 x as a many repetitions as possible*
- *Dumbbell Deadlift – 3 x 15 repetitions*
- *Resistance Band Overhead Shoulder Press – 3 x 15 repetitions*
- *Fitness Ball Wheelbarrow*
- *Alternating Dumbbell Curls – 2 x 12*
- *Suspension Swimmer Pull – 2 x 12*
- *Skipping 3 x 30 seconds (as fast as possible)*

The Basement Gym

If you are fortunate enough to have a dedicated space in which to house a permanent gym, then you have the ability to create a training facility to rival anything you'd see in a commercial gym. The quality of the gear provided in the home gym market has improved drastically in the last 10 years. You can now buy equipment that is as solid and durable as that used in commercial gyms, but for a fraction of the price.

Here's your essential equipment list for your basement gym:

✓ <u>Power Rack</u>

- ✓ Multi function bench
- ✓ Olympic Bar
- ✓ Plates
- ✓ TRX Suspension System
- ✓ Exercise Mat
- ✓ Skipping Rope

Power Rack

A power rack will form the foundation piece of any decent basement gym. It consists of a cage like device, which is designed to allow a person to exercise with heavy weight safely with having to rely on another person to act as a 'spotter.' The rack looks like a walk in metal cube, made up of four uprights that are joined by horizontal cross-beams. The end uprights have a series of holes for safety catches to sit at various heights. There are also j-cups for the lifting bar to sit on.

A power rack will afford you the benefit of safety, rigidity and versatility. Inside a power rack you can perform an endless number of movements confidently and safely, including:

- ✓ Squats
- ✓ Deadlifts

- ✓ Bench press
- ✓ Up right rowing
- ✓ Shrugs
- ✓ Inverted rows
- ✓ Pull ups
- ✓ Dips
- ✓ Rack pulls
- ✓ Barbell curls

Here's what to look for in a power rack . . .

- ➢ **Hole spacing** – the hole spacing on the uprights will determine how well you are able to personalize the bar position to your body. Many racks only offer a two-inch gap. This is ok for squats but, when it comes to upper body exercises like the bench press, you need it to close up to one inch. The Westside spacing system does just that; it has two inch gaps at the top and bottom of the rack, closing to one inch through the central region – look out for it.

- ➢ **Secure Pins** – Your safety pins are the things that will catch the weight if you fail during a lift, so they need to be reliable. Thick steel construction and secure locking are non negotiable.

➤ **Dimensions** – Measure out your available space, including the maximum height available. When sizing up a rack, remember to include space for the bar to over hang on each side of the rack. You'll also need room to work in the area at changing and securing weight plates. Think, too, about the maximum height. You will need to make allowance for head height above the bar when doing pull ups.

➤ **Construction** – Power racks are designed for lifting heavy weight so they need to be made to last. Set as your minimum standard, 11 gauge, 2 x 3 inch steel with five eighth inch bolts and fasteners.

➤ **Pull Up Bar attachment** – Most power racks will feature a pull up bar. Make sure that the one you select offers a range of grip options, including neutral grip and extra wide.

Multi Function Bench

A weight bench provides the platform for a lot of the work that you will be doing in your home gym, especially when you are working with dumbbells. There are three types of bench that you can purchase as follows:

1) Bench Station – this type of bench comes with a built in stand for a weight bar to sit on.

2) Standard flat bench – a low-lying, non-adjustable flat bench.

3) Utility Bench – adjustable for flat, incline or decline work.

The best type of bench that will give you the most options is a utility bench. Here are 5 things go consider when looking for a utility bench . . .
   ✓ Maximum weight rating (you'll want at least 400 lbs.)
   ✓ Pad firmness
   ✓ Bench height
   ✓ Bench width

You really need to test drive a bench to see if the firmness, height and width work for you. In terms of height, you don't want it too high that you can't plant your feet firmly on the floor when exercising. If it's too low you'll be prevented from getting into position to exert maximum force when lifting. A bench that is too wide will not allow for proper flexion of the lats when doing exercises such as dumbbell flyes.

Barbell

Barbells may all look the same, but there are some distinct differences between them. When you're shopping for a bar you want something that will see you through a lifetime of training. Here's what to look out for . . .

> ➢ Strength – you need a bar that can handle up to 1000 lbs, is 7 feet long and weighs 45 lbs.

> ➢ Sleeves – revolving sleeves allow you to perform a wider range of movements, including the Olympic lifts.

> ➢ Knurling – the knurled part that you grip allows for a stronger hold. But you don't want it too knurled or your hands will tear up.

Plates

You can pick up cheap plates second hand if you wish. After all, a weight is a weight. But there are some advantages to buying new. Buying plates that are coated in heavy-duty rubber will make them far more resilient. They'll also be a lot safer when dropped – and much quieter.

Sample Basement Gym Workout Program

Monday and Thursday
  - ➤ *Warm Up – 5 mins skipping*
  - ➤ *Squats – 3 x 12 repetitions*
  - ➤ *Suspension Rear Lunges – 3 x 15 repetitions*
  - ➤ *Pull Ups – 3 x as many as possible*
  - ➤ *Suspension T-Pull – 2 x 12*
  - ➤ *Suspended Plank – 3 x 20 seconds*

Tuesday and Friday
  - ➤ *Warm Up - 5 mins skipping*
  - ➤ *Deadlift – 3 x 12 repetitions*
  - ➤ *Bench Press – 3 x 12 repetitions*
  - ➤ *Suspension Flyes 3 x 12 repetitions*
  - ➤ *Barbell Curls – 3 x 12 repetitions*

> ➤ *Suspension Triceps Extension – 3 x 12 repetitions*
> ➤ *Suspension Knee Tucks – 3 x 15*

Keeping Fit While Travelling

You've been doing an awesome job of keeping your workouts regular. You haven't missed your after work sweat sessions for months and it feels great. But now, you've got a week long work trip out of town.

Looks like your training schedule is about to fly out the window and all of your hard work is about to be undone.

Actually, there's no reason why a work trip need curtail your workout schedule. With a little planning and some good old fashioned determination you can actually allow your change of scenery to spice up and complement, rather than derail, your training program. Here are half a dozen ways to keep fit while working away.

1) Utilize the hotel gym - Though most hotels do have a gymnasium, many of them are rather sparsely equipped. With a bit of forward

planning, however, you wil be able to stick to your training routine. Check their website ahead of time to see what facilities they have. If it's not much more than a room with a rower and weight stack, consider purchasing a DVD workout, such as Insanity, and take your laptop to the gym with you

2) Train in Your Room - All you need for a terrific work-out is a 1 meter square space. Start with high knee jogging for 1 minute, followed by butt kicks and then sprinting in place, for a total 3 minute warm-up. Move into a giant set of push-ups, the plank, wall sits, body-weight squats and reverse dips. Repeat for 5 sets.

3) Use the Pool - Doing laps in the hotel pool is a great way to revitalize your training. It'll give you a great cardiovascular workout as well as working your shoulders and core to the max. Give yourself a challenging number and keep going until you hit it!

4) Check out the Scenery - Pack your trainers and go for a twilight jog while taking in the sights of your work location. If work is going to keep you up late, pound the pavement early in the morning. If this is the only training you'll be doing, drop after every 500 meters and pump out 25 pushups.

5) Find a local commercial gym - Training in a new gym can be a real treat. Often you'll find new and different pieces of equipment to train on. It's a great way to revitalize your training and meet new people. If you're lucky you may even find a local branch of your gym at home where you'll be able to train for free.

6) Keep Your Nutrition Strict - Well, semi-strict anyway. If you're going to reach for a pastry, make sure that it's just one. Go for the salad bar, the lean proteins and fish. Desserts don't have to be sugar laden. Choose the fruit salads and Angel cake. And don't go

overboard on the alcohol - it, too, is full of calories.

Home Cardio

The debate over the most effective form of aerobic exercise has been raging ever since Dr Kenneth Cooper coined the term 'Aerobics' in the early 70's. Today, there are two diametrically opposed groups – those who advocate slow state, steady cardio and others who swear by high intensity, short duration cardio sessions. When it comes to fat loss, the truth lies somewhere in the middle. Here are 14 tips to allow you to get the most out of both exercise types without having to step foot into a gym . . .

Tip No. 1: Hit it Hard and Fast with HIIT Training

How To Do It: Choose a cardio exercise that you can do go all out on (running, cycling, rowing, etc). After a warm-up, sprint for 20 seconds at absolute max capacity. Then walk for precisely 10 seconds. Repeat for 7 more cycles.

Why Do It: High Intensity Interval Training (HIIT) not only burns more calories than slow state cardio, it also boosts your metabolism, allowing your body to burn more calories all day long. It also allows you to get in an awesome workout in a short period of time.

When to do it: Perform your HIIT training every second day. On alternate days, do your weight training workout.

Tip No. 2: Don't do your HIIT cardio on an empty stomach

How To Do It: Get some fast acting carbs in your body to fuel you through your HIIT session by way of a banana or two or a pre-workout drink.

Why Do It: HIIT training requires energy. Energy comes from food. If you were to do your HIIT training on an empty stomach you negatively will impact upon your efficiency.

When to do it: 15 minutes prior to doing your HIIT cardio.

Tip No. 3: Run on the sand

How To Do It: Take yourself down to the beach and go for a jog along the water's edge. Then do a series of sprints before diving in for a well-deserved swim.

Why Do It: Running on the sand takes a whole lot more energy than running on a hard surface. That means that you'll be burning more calories – and giving your calves a fantastic workout.

When to do it: Once a week, mix it up a little by heading to the beach.

Tip No. 4: Mix up the intensity on the treadmill

How To Do It: Alternate sixty-second periods of intense sprinting with sixty seconds of medium to low intensity work.

When To Do It: You won't burn fat by walking on the treadmill for an hour while reading your Ipad. By switching back and forth between maximum intensity and medium pace training, you'll be revving up the metabolism and improving your heart health.

When to do it: Every time you jump on the treadmill, which should happen on the days that you don't do your HIIT training.

Tip No. 5: Know your heart rate training zone

How To Do It: Find your ideal training heart rate with the following calculation . . .

220 – your age x 75%

Why Do It: Training within your heart rate zone allows you to work optimally, burning the most calories and receiving the most cardiovascular benefit.

When to do it: When you're doing your non-HIIT cardio training. While doing HIIT just go as fast as you possibly can – you won't have time to worry about your heart rate!

Tip No. 6: Buy a pedometer and use it

How To Do It: Purchase a good pedometer, clip it on and make sure that you get a minimum of 10,000 steps every day. All of the steps you do every day counts. If that's not enough, top it up with a power walk.

Why do it: Your non-exercise movement counts. In fact, incorporating more activity into your daily routine is the goal of life line fitness – and this is a great way to make sure that you are doing just that.

When to do it: Every day – 10,000 steps before you can go to bed!

Tip No. 7: Mix up your cardio

How To Do It: Within a cardio session, rather than 45 minutes on one machine, choose 3 machines and do 15 minutes on each. As an example you could work on the treadmill, elliptical machine and a rowing machine.

Why Do It: A change in cardio is a great way to break through a fat loss plateau. It also helps to stave off boredom. Mixing it up also allows you to work a range of stabilizer muscles and takes the strain off joints that may be caused from prolonged movement through one plane.

When to do it: Every couple of weeks, completely change around your cardio choices. Within a single workout, do shorter sessions on a variety of machines.

Tip No. 8: Boot Camp it

How To Do It: Sign up to a boot camp, kickboxing or circuit-training class.

When To Do It: By performing body weight exercises and conditioning drills non-stop or in circuits, the workout becomes cardiovascular in nature. The calorie burn is also very high. These classes are often a good fit for people who don't gel with cardio machines.

When to do it: Typically boot camp type classes happen twice a week, with two days between each session.

Tip No. 9: Run Up Stairs

How To Do It: Find a place where you can run up a flight of between 30 and 50 steps. Start with a warm up jog and then sprint up and walk down. Repeat this 10 to 12 times. If you can't find any stairs to climb, hill running comes in a close second.

Why Do It: Runing stairs is a fantatsic way to rmp up your cardio sessions. It will give you a fantastic cardio workout, burn a ton of calories –and it will provide an amazing leg pump.

When to do it: Try stair running once a week to add variety and intensity to your program.

Tip No. 10: Do your cardio first thing in the morning

How To Do It: Set your alarm clock to allow you to get your cardio in before the rest of your day kicks in.

Why Do It: Taking positive action early in the morning starts your day on the right foot and makes you feel good all day long. Training after work, when you're exhausted and distracted by the issues of the day makes it more likely that you'll skip your workout.

When to do it: 7 am, 6 am, 5 am ??? The busier you are, the earlier you'll have to get up – all you have to do is overcome mind over mattress syndrome.

Tip No. 11: Do moderate intensity cardio on an empty stomach

How To Do It: Get straight into your early morning moderate intensity cardio training without no food. Drink plenty of water, however, and have a 50 percent carbohydrate and 30 percent protein meal about 30 minutes after your session finishes.

When To Do It: Cardio on an empty stomach allows fat to be more easily released from fat cells and burned for energy.

Who is it ideal for: People who are doing moderate intensity cardio only in the morning. If you are following it with weight training, you're better off getting some fuel into your system.

Tip No. 12: Utilize cardio periodization

How To Do It: Cycle the intensity and duration of your cardio to prevent burn out and overtraining.

Why Do It: Intense cardio day after day, without let up, is too stressful on the body. By doing so, you run the risk of mental and physical burn out.

When to do it: Every 6 weeks, take a one weeks break from cardio, then spend two weeks just doing low to moderate intensity before starting the next high intensity cycle.

Tip No. 13: Try Kettlebell Cardio

How To Do It: Grab a kettle bell and start performing two handle kettlebell swings for a set of 20 reps. Then do a set of push ups. Now go back to the kettlebell swings. Do six cycles of this superset for a fantastic workout which improves your VO2 max while churning through the calories.

Why Do It: As well as providing a great calorie burning workout, kettlebells are an excellent way to improve your functional fitness. In other words, they work your muscles in a similar way to how they work during your everyday activities.

When to do it: Throw in a kettlebell session every couple of weeks to add some variety to your cardio routine.

Tip No. 14: Carry Extra weight while doing your cardio

How To Do It: Wear a weight vest or ankle weights while performing your cardio sessions.

Why Do It: Carrying extra weight during cardio has been proven to improve fast twitch muscle fiber recruitment, as well as calorie burning and recovery.

When to do it: Slowly start adding weight to one cardio session per week – just make sure that the added resistance doesn't deter from your exercise performance.

Chapter 4: Exercising at the Gym

As beneficial as setting up a home gym is, some people simply prefer the atmosphere of a gym. Of course, there are also many who cannot afford the initial outlay of setting up a home gym or just have no inclination to buy their own equipment. There's also the fact that a commercial gym will always have more training variety and is able to offer group classes and personal training. Whatever the reason, if your choice is to sign up for a gym membership, then this chapter is for you.

Getting Started at the Gym

Once you've signed up at a gym, you need to figure out the best time for you to train. This will obviously depend on your schedule. If possible, it would pay to attend outside of the busy zones, which are between 6:30 and 8:00 am and 4:30 and 7:00 pm.

You should have a pre exercise meal at least 30 minutes before going to the gym. You need food in your body when you that the gym that will do the following:

- ✓ Provide energy for your training session
- ✓ Protect and preserve your muscle mass
- ✓ Enhance muscle growth

Here are 4 meal ideas that will deliver those results;
1) Oatmeal
2) Hard boiled eggs with an avocado salad
3) Grilled chicken (6 oz.) with sweet potato

It is vital, also that you stay well hydrated during your workout. Always take a water bottle with you and sip from it between sets.

You'll need a gym bag, which should contain your change of clothes for after your post workout shower, a towel, a lock for your gym locker and your personal grooming items.

You need to go out and buy a new wardrobe to go to the gym. But you will need to wear training shoes (most gyms will not let you train in bare feet for safety reasons). You don't want to wear clothes that are too tight. Ideally loose fitting fabric that is able to breathe is the best choice. Certain gyms will not let you train in a tank top or a singlet so check out the requirement so you don't get embarrassed.

Gym Etiquette

Gym etiquette is an essential part of the shared training experience.

Here are the basic common sense rules that you need to follow:

> Training right in front of the dumbbell rack – simply step back to allow other people access to the weights to give everyone else free access to the rack.
> Taking up more space than you need – don't spread your personal around the gym and do not hog benches that you're not using.
> Interrupting someone in the middle of their set – respect their space and their focus.
> Return your weights to the rack when you're done.

- ➤ Check that machines and benches are free if you are unsure.
- ➤ Wipe down equipment when you're done.
- ➤ Stay home of you're sick – don't spread your germs.
- ➤ Don't do curls in the squat rack.
- ➤ Don't blast music – use headphones.
- ➤ Don't over socialize at the gym
- ➤ Un-rack weights when you've finished with a machine or a bar.

Why You Need to Be Training With Weights

- ➤ Training with weights burns a whole lot of calories
- ➤ Training with weights boost your metabolism
- ➤ Training with weights allows you to sculpt, shape and build your body
- ➤ Training with weights gets you strong
- ➤ Training with weights will make you aerobically fit
- ➤ Training with weights builds muscle
- ➤ Training with weights churns through body fat

> Training with weights enhances bone density
> Training with weights develops self esteem and self discipline

The 10 Commandments of Weight Training

Gym training is primarily about resistance or weight training. The following 10 commandments will give you a heads start on the smart way to pump iron.

1) **Specificity**. If you want to compete on the Mr Olympia stage you are going to train a whole lot differently than a house wife who's focused on firmingher middle after her 3rd baby. That's the principle of specificity. A specific result requires a specific training program. You therefore, are using the weights as a tool to achieve your ends. An example of the principle of specificity in action could relate to a basketball player. The principle dictates that the exercises he chooses will mimic what he does on the court. For

legs, he can choose squats or he can choose leg extensions. Squats more closely mimic the jumping movements required in basketball, whereas leg extensions are an isolation exercise. The basketball player would choose to do squats.

2) **Overload**. The overload principle means that you need to be constantly lifting more weight, performing more repetitions or decreasing your between set rest than you did during your last workout.

3) **Progressive Resistance.** This principle dates way back to Milo of Croton, a 6th century, BCE wrestler. Legend tells us that, as a boy, Milo started carrying a newborn calf every day as it grew to maturity. The calf got heavier every day, but, because the increments were so small, Milo didn't notice them. By the time the bull had grown to maturity, Milo was able to carry it around his family farm. Weight trainers have been drawing inspiration from Milo ever since. By increasing the

weight by small increments each workout, you'll be able to dramatically improve your strength, which will enhance your intensity and boost your fat loss results.

4) **Intensity.** Intensity relates to the amount of effort you put into your training sessions. When you're doing an exercise, you'll want the last couple of reps tp be very hard – to the oint where you couldn't do another rep with proper form. If you finish a set and you feel like you could perform another 2 or 3 reps then you are not working at sufficient intensity. You need to either increase the weight, increase the reps or decrease the rest between each set.

5) **Rep Range.** Rep range relates to the number of times that you perform a movement. To get the most out of your training you need to ensure that you are using the ideal number of reps for your specific training goal. The traditional rep ranges are as follows:

> ➤ 4 to 7 reps for strength
> ➤ 8-12 reps for building muscle
> ➤ 13-20 reps for fat loss and endurance

6) **Volume.** Volume relates to the number of sets and reps required for optimal training. This is an area of much debate, with advocates of extremely low volume training (one set per exercise) citing scientific studies to support their view just as passionately as those who swear by high volume training (20 sets per body part). The ideal training volume is in between those extremes. 3-4 sets per working set seems to be about ideal.

7) **Rest.** The period of time that you rest between sets is critical. It can range from very short (30 seconds) to very long (3 minutes +). You need enough time to recover from the last set just enough to allow for a full out effort on the next one. If you wait too long before starting the next set, you won't be able to build your

intensity level.. You want to build from one set to the next. For that reason you will rest for 60 seconds between each set.

8) **Tempo.** The speed tht oit tkes to complete your repetitions is very important. On every repetition, you perform a positive part (lifting) and a negative part (lowering). When you lift a resistance, you are shortening the muscle. When you lower it, the muscle gets longer.. It is imperative that you use a controlled tempo which allows you to isolate the working muscle and avoid momentum in the lift. The lowering, or negative part, of the exercise should take twice as long as the lifting, or positive part. It should take you 2 seconds to lift, and 4 seconds to lower it. Doing it slower resists gravity and increases intensity.

9) **Variation.** Periodically changing your workout program prevents your body from becoming accustomed to the workload that is being placed upon it. This helps to

avoid training plateaus and keeps your body guessing and responding. It also prevents training boredom and allows you to work your body from a variety of angles. You should change your program every six weeks.

10)   **Recuperation.** When you work out, you are placing stress on your body. **You are depleting your reserves of energy, breaking down muscle tissue and putting you in a state of fatigue.** It is after the workout that recovery and rebuilding takes place. That's why you need 48 hours rest between workouts.

Two Key Functional Weight Training Principles

1) Balanced Development Around Joints:

At each joint, muscle groups work against one another in pairs to provide stability, much like guy-wires on opposite sides of a tent pole.

Most day-to-day movements involves these muscle pairs working together. When you rock a heavy piece of furniture back and forth to move it, you are using several several of these pairings; at the elbow, triceps to push, biceps to pull; at the shoulder, anterior deltoid and pecs to push, posterior deltoids and back to pull; and at the waist, abdominals and spinal erectors working against one another to stabilize the body. Balanced development requires devoting equal effort to developing these opposing muscle groups. Only with a balanced approach will you achieve true functional strength. In the process you will develop a symmetrically proportioned body while staving off muscular imbalance injuries.

2) **Train From the Ground Up**:

In training from the ground up, you will train your legs before your upper body. Here's why:

You should train with the most important exercises first. Your legs are involved in more daily activities than any other muscle group - both directly (running, walking) and indirectly (providing stability for upper body movements). The legs also play an important role in circulation. Although your heart pumps blood through the arteries out to the rest of your body, there is no organ responsible for pumping blood back to the heart. Pumping action is supplied by movement of the muscles, especially the large muscles in the legs. By focusing first on legs when you are freshest, then, you will be supporting better blood return and a healthier, more powerful circulatory system.

Leave Your Ego at the Door

You see them in every gym. Guys who are hanging around the heavy weight equipment - usually the bench press - intent on pushing as much weight as they can. No, they're not powerlifters. In fact, judging by their form, they're not weight lifters at all. They'll use anything short of a wheel jack to get the weight up. Grunting, contorting, lifting their hips and back off the bench, these guys are the epitome of bad form. But they don't care - as long as they bench 300.

You can't learn much from these clowns. What you can learn is to get rid of your ego before you walk into the gym. You are there to give your body the best workout of it's life - the workout that will maximize fat loss and sculpt your body ideal. Now, here's the thing. . .

Your muscle has no idea how heavy the weight is.

The only thing that registers with your muscle is how intensely has to work. Those guys on the bench press - despite throwing a lot of weight around - are not working their target muscle group (the pectorals) very hard at all. All of the work is being achieved through hip thrust and momentum. In doing so, they are risking major injury.

The take home message here is that the weight is a tool to work your muscles, nothing more, nothing less. And, just as a builder doesn't wax lyrical about the beauty of his hammer, you'd be silly to focus on the weight at the expense of form.

Many people are surprised when they see professional bodybuilders working out with much lighter weights than they would have imagined. These people know that the weight on the bar is just one way to achieve maximum intensity. They are using the weight as a tool and have learnt to leave their ego behind. So should you.

Should I Hire a Personal Trainer?

When you join a gym, you'll no doubt be offered the services of a personal trainer. The trainer will train you on a one-on-one basis. You can arrange a package to suit your budget and your requirements where they either work with you every single workout, once per week or less frequently than that.

Personal trainers are quite expensive. You can expect to pay anything from $30 to $150 per session. So, what are the advantages of hiring a personal trainer?

✓ A personal trainer will teach you how to use the gym equiment, set up a balanced schedule to maximize your time and get the best out of your workout.

- ✓ A personal trainer will teach you correct exercise form and monitor your form as youe exercise.
- ✓ A personla trainer will inspire and motivate you to progress toward your goals.
- ✓ A personal trainer will push you past your self imposed limits to get the most out of your workout

It may noy be within your budget to hire a personal trainer long term. Still, it is a good idea to have at least a couple of sessions with a trainer when you first start at the gym so that you learn proper exercise technique.

Intensity Enhancers

Once you've been training with weights for about six months, you will be in a position to step up your training intensity. This will allow you to continue making progress and counter the natural plateuing of progress that will occur as your body gets used to your workout routine. The following 5 techniques will allow you to up the intensity and keep the gains coming.

Forced Reps

An ideal set involves finding ways to vary the amount of reistance as the set progresses. This will allow you to work with maximum intensity on every rep. There are several ways to get the amount of weight to vary like that. The simplest is with forced reps.

Forced reps are performed when your training partner assists you to perform the last two or three reps of a set. They provide just enough help to allow you complete the set with good form.

For example:

Let's say the amount of weight you can bench press is 185 pounds. Your average set goes like this: the first two or three reps at this weight are easily within your ability, the fourth starts to get pretty hard, the fifth and sixth are really hard and you can just barely do the seventh and eighth.

Next set, you can barely do five reps. Third set you can barely do three.

Normally, you might drop the weight during second and third sets to allow you to get out the required six to eight reps. However, the point remains that you can do the first few reps, even in these later sets. The weight isn't too heavy, it's just that your strength has diminished due to the work you've already done.

With a partner to help you, however, you can use the higher weight for all three (or four) sets, and have the partner "adjust" the amount of weight you are pushing to match your decreasing strength.

For each set you would do as many as possible unassisted. When you are unable to complete a rep by yourself, your training partner gives just enough assistance to cmplete the repetition.

Keep in mind that forced reps is an advanced technique and is much more intense than doing normal reps. It's also more dangerous. If your partner looks away at the wrong moment or jerks the weights when you're on your last strength reserve, you could be severely injured. Do forced reps only with a partner you trust.

Partial Reps

Partial reps are just what they sound like. They involve finishing off an exercise by doing only a part of the full range of motion associated with that exercise.

For example, suppose you're doing dips. When you reach the point at which you would normally not be able to press yourself up to the starting position if you went down all the way, you would squeeze out a few more reps just going down part way.

Super-sets

Super-sets involve performing two exercises consecutively with no rest between them. The exercises may be for the same body part or they may be for opposing muscles groups, such as biceps and triceps.

An example of a super-set for the same body part is doing a set of barbell curls and then immediately performing a set of close grip pull ups, both of which target the biceps.

An example of a superset for opposing muscle groups is doing a set of barbell curls and then doing a set of lying triceps extensions.

An opposing muscle group is one that works in the opposite direction to another muscle group. When one muscle group is pushing, the opposite muscle group is pulling. The opposing muscle groups in your body are . . .

Pectorals / Latissimus Dorsi

Biceps / Triceps
Abdominals / Spinal Erectors

Quadriceps / Hamstrings

Giant Sets
Giant sets consist of a series of exercises for the sae body part that are done consecutively with no rest between them. Often the exercises target different portions of the same muscle groups, such as the anterior, posterior and medial heads of the shoulders.

Pyramiding

Pyramiding relates to the weight and repetitions of the set you are doing. With each succeeding set, you increase the weight and decrease the number fo repetitions. This technique is most applicable to compound movements that enhance functional strength.

Here's ane example of how you might pyramid your bench press . . .

Set One 12 reps x 150 lbs
Set Two 10 reps x 160 lbs
Set Three 8 reps x 165 lbs
Set four 6 reps x 170 lbs

Pre-Exhaustion

Often when you are working a torso muscle group, such as the chest or back, you will find that your smaller muscle groups which are involved in the lift, such as the triceps, will give up before you have maximally worked the target muscle group.

This creates a problem . . .

How can you work the target muscle to the max when your smaller muscle group gives out before your target muscle does? The solution is wrapped up in the technique known as pre-exhaution.

Here's how it works . . .

Taking the example of the chest as the target muscle group, your main exercise is the dumbbell bench press. Firstly, however, you perform a set of flat bench dumbbell flyes. This exercise targets the chest muscles, without really stimulating the triceps. When you've completed 12 reps of flyes, go directly to the dumbbell bench press.

Because, you have already pre-exhausted your chest, they become the weak link during your main exercise. This means that they will give out before the triceps, allowing your chest to receive maximum stimulation.

The key to success with this technique is to move directly from the first exercise to the second with absolutely no rest. Set up both sets of dumbbells ahead of time. You will also find that the weight you use on the second exercise will go down. That doesn't matter. Remember, all that the target muscle knows is how hard it is beng worked, and pre-exhaustion will allow you to work it a whole lot harder.

Descending Sets

Descending sets involves doing four to six sets of an exercise with no rest. The normal rep range is between 6 and 8. On each succeeding set you reduce the weight slightly. The easiest way to perform descending sets is by standing in front of a rack of dumbbells. Start with the heaviest weight that you can handle for 6 reps. Grasp the weights and perform your 6 strict reps. Now place the weights back in the rack and grasp hold of the next set going down the rack. Perform another six reps. Keep working down the rack until you have completed your required number of sets.

Descending (or strip) sets can also be performed with a barbell. Ideally, you'll need two spotters. If you are doing the bench press, start with a weight that will allow you to eek out 6 reps. Then rack the bar as your partners strip 5 pounds off each end of the bar. Now pump out another six reps. Continue this process, going down in gradations of 5 pounds each time.

Gym Cardio

One of the first things that you'll notice when you walk into any gym is the number of treadmills and eliptical trainers in the place. You'll see people strolling away on them, as if they were out for a Sunday walk in the park, while hardly breaking a sweat at all. What they are doing is known as steady state cardio. It is low intensity, long duration aerobic exercise that never lifts their heart rate above 65% of their maximum (to find your maximum heart rate, subtract your age from 220).

Steady state cardio is not the most efficient use of your gym time.

The reason?

It is not intense enough.

You've already learnt about the importantce of training intensity and the same principle applies to cardio training. The best way to achieve it is with High Intensity Interval Training (HIIT). HIIT involves performing short bursts of hard and fast cardio followed by brief rest periods. The cycle is repeated a number of times.

HIIT has been the subject of many clinical studies. Here are the proven benefits:

- ➤ It takes far less time to perform
- ➤ You can perform HIIT wthout any equipment
- ➤ HIIT increases your aerobic capacity more effectively than steady state cardio
- ➤ HIIT increases your lactic threshold, meaning that it can better handle the build up of lactic acid in your muscles
- ➤ HIIT improves insulin sensitvity, a key fat loss determinant
- ➤ HIIT can boost testosterone and growth hormone levels to enahnce muscle growth
- ➤ HIIT burns more calories than steady state cardio
- ➤ HIIT revs up your metabolsim so you're burning calories throughout the day

You can perform HIIT using virtualy any type of cardio equipment. In the gym you can do it with . . .

> A treadmill
> A rowing machine
> A skipping rope
> Burpees

Here's an example using the treadmill:

Do a 5 minute warm-up at a low speed of between 3 and 4 miles per hour. As you hit the 4:30 mark, start increasing the speed until it is at a challenging running speed for you when the timer reaches 5 minutes. Now sprint for 20 seconds, going as hard as you possibly can. As soon as 20 srconds is up, jump your feet to the side rails fo the treadmill and rest for 10 seconds. Then immediatley jump back on and sprint for another 20 seconds. Repeat this pattern until you have completed 8 sprints. Then bring the speed back down to between 3 and 4 miles per hour and finish with a 5 minute warm down.

You should perform HIIT training 3 times per week on alternate days. For the sake of variety, change up the apparatus you use each time.

Circuit Training

As great as HIIT is, there are times when your body needs variety. That is why you should alternate 6 weeks of HIIT training with 6 weeks of weights based circuit training. This will allow you to add variety while upping the cardiovascular effect of some of the exercises that you will be used to performing in your regular weight training program. The following program will allow you to capitalize on the gains made from your main workout program while improving your cardiovascular fitness and overall appearance.

Do your circuit training on the days that you don't do your regular weights session, but only on 2 days per week. On the third day, you can add in a HIIT session - that's up to you.

Circuit training is a bit like musical chairs. You, along with other trainers in your gym, start at a given exercise station. A light flashes for 15 seconds.

For the next minute you perform strict repetitions of that exercise. After a minute the light flashes for another 15 seconds. You now have that long to get in position for the next exercise, ready to start before the light stops flashing. Now you perform a minute's worth of reps on that station. During a half hour workout, you will perform 30 exercises. This will not only give you an effective acrdio workout, it will also work every muscle in your body.

Here are 4 key reasons why you should incorporate circuit training into your routine:

1. Circuit training increases your strength, hitting every muscle in the body
2. Circuit training burns a whole lot of calories
3. Circuit training improves your cardiovascular fitness
4. Circuit training adds variety to your workouts

Circuit Essentials

➢ Even though your gym may have already have a circuit laid out, you can easily add in exercises. If they haven't alternated a weights exercise (Lat pull-downs) with an aerobic exercise (Prisoner Squats), then throw some aerobic moves in to mix it up.

➢ Choose a lighter weight than normal - one that allows you to perform about 30 reps within the minute.

➢ Don't get out of sequence - if you do, you will annoy everyone else who's doing the circuit.

Design Your Own Fat Burning Workout

You don't have to rely on others to lead you by the hand when it comes to knowing how to train. Follow these 6 easy steps to designing your own mega fat burning workout.

Step One: Compound the Fat Burn

Create an exercise circuit that revolves around compound exercises that work a number of muscle groups together, such as squats, deadlifts and barbell rows. Why compound movements? An exercise like squats engages a number of muscles at once - thighs, glutes, calves, abs and lower back, to name a few. This means that it burns more calories and increases your workout intensity over a shorter period of time. On the other hand, exercise that involve only one muscle group, such as barbell curls, don't require as much energy.

Step Two: Go Heavy

A lot of people make the mistake of using very light weights for 15 reps or more, with the thought that more reps will help burn calories and body **fat. It won't.** Muscle tissue burns fat - and the best way to build muscle is to use sets of 8 - 12 reps. The weight should be heavy enough that you're challenged to finish the set.

Step Three: Keep It Short

You don't need two hours in the gym every day to achieve your dream body. About 30 minutes of focused weight room exercise is all you need, coupled with 20 minutes of cardio.Rest for only as long as it takes to move between exercises in the middle of circuits. Stay focused on the task at hand and work intensely.

Step Four: Get a Minimum of Two Workouts a Week

To lose fat, you're going to have to put forth a little effort. Two weight training and cardio workouts a week is the minimum, three is closer to ideal. If circuit training is your thing, then you'll have to create two upper body and two lower body circuits. Include three exercises per week.

Step Five: Use Intervals for Cardio

You can get an incredible cardio workout in
20 minutes by harnessing the power of intervals. Sprint for 20 seconds every minute. Simply watch the timer and between 30 seconds and 50 seconds of every minute, crank up the machine to a sprint. For the remaining time within each minute, jog at a slower pace.

Step Six: Evaluate Your Progress Regularly

After six weeks on your self designed program, stop and evaluate your progress. If positive changes to your body weren't taking place, stop and rethink your strategy. Don't settle for zero progress. Change it up within the parameters outlined above and dig in for another six weeks.

Sample Circuit Routine

Upper Body Circuit One:

Military Press
Bench Press
Close Grip Bench Press

Upper Body Circuit Two:

Bent Over Barbell Row
Seated Cable Row
Pull Up

Lower Body Circuit One:

Body Weight Squat
Barbell Hack Squat
Deadlift

Lower Body Circuit Two:
Barbell Squat

Lunge
Single Leg Romanian Deadlift

Do upper body circuits one day, lower body another. If you want to work out three days a week, go back to upper body on your next training day and continue the pattern. Run through each circuit two or three times, performing 8 - 12 reps of each exercise per circuit.

Gym Training Checklist

- ➤ Use HIIT training as your cardio mainstay 3 x per week
- ➤ Every six weeks switch your cardio to circuit training
- ➤ Use progressive resistance to increase the intensity of each succeeding workout
- ➤ Rest for 30 seconds between sets
- ➤ Use a 2 second up, 4 second down training tempo
- ➤ Change your workout program every six weeks
- ➤ Allow 48 hours between working a muscle group
- ➤ Ensure balanced development around joints
- ➤ Train from the center of your body out

- ➢ Train from the ground up
- ➢ Focus on compound, functional exercises
- ➢ Always keep your core tight and your back flat when holding a weight
- ➢ Always use a closed grip when grasping a bar
- ➢ Never use momentum to lift a weight
- ➢ Leave your ego at the door

Chapter 5: Maintaining the Momentum

You have now gotten yourself off the couch and into the exercise mode.

That's great.

The challenge now is to maintain that momentum. The last thing you want is to be another one of those people who jump in with all guns blazing, only to crash and burn after three weeks. No, you want exercise to be a daily habit that becomes a vital part of your lifestyle. In this chapter, you'll discover 15 tactics that you can implement to make exercise your newest and greatest habit.

Tactic #1: Focus on your end goal every day. Write it out as a positive statement tied to a date and stick it to your mirror. Here's an example . . .

On May 1ˢᵗ, 2016 I will be at 20% body fat.

Tactic #2: Take in Fitness Knowledge. There is a vast amount of information at your fingertips relating to exercise. The more you educate yourself, the more motivated you'll become. Learn about all of the different forms of exercise, from yoga to pilates, stretching to weight training. Each form of exercise has it's unique aspects and benefits. Learn how you can make the most of them.

Tactic #3: Use Habit Anchoring. Habit anchoring involves committing yourself to a very small change of habits that is attached to something that you already do. Make positive affirmations to yourself relating to the anchor and the habit. Here's an example . . .

After I get into my car after work, I will drive straight to the gym.

Tactic #4: Make Mini Commitments. Commit yourself to exercising 30 minutes each day for 20 days in a row. Make the commitment small and manageable.

Tactic #5: Get Rid of Obstacles to Exercise. There will always be a nagging voice in your mind that will look for obstacles to working out. You have to be prepared in order to defeat those obstacles. The first thing you should do is to set out everything you need for your workout the evening before. If you're going to the gym, have your workout clothing, your shower items and change of clothing, water bottle and sweat towel ready to go. If you are training at home, have everything set out and ready to train.

Tactic #6: Make it Enjoyable. Never allow yourself to get bored when exercising. Keep your workouts interesting by joining group fitness classes, experiment with different types of exercise, different styles of workout and different exercise modes. Every now and again find a new workout location, jump on a different machine or take part in a workout competition.

Tactic #7: Use Technology. Technology can help you to monitor, keep on top of and stay motivated with your workout. Products like the *Fitbit* will also provide you with some friendly competition.

Tactic #8: Make Yourself Accountable. Tell others about your commitment to regular exercise. Doing so will provide you with external sources of motivation to keep going. When you share your goals with your family and friends, you know that they are going to check back with you to see how you are going. That will keep you accountable.

Tactic #9: Don't Be Discouraged by Lack of Visible Results. A lot of people feel discouraged when they don't see the scale weight coming down after working our for a few weeks. That's often because they have gained a bit of muscle while losing fat. Because muscle weighs five times more than fat, the scale weight won't drop – it may in fact go up slightly. The key is to focus on developing the habit of regular exercise. The changes will come in time.

Tactic #10: Anticipate Plateaus. After a couple of months of working out, your results are bound to slow down or even stop altogether for a period of time. This is perfectly natural. It is because your body has adapted to the new stresses that you are imposing upon it. To overcome these plateaus, change up your training every six weeks. This will keep your body guessing and responding.

Tactic #11: Face Up To Self Limiting Beliefs. That negative voice will throw up doubts that designed to get you to question every positive step you're taking. It will question the point of working out, try to convince you that the plan won't work, remind you that you've failed at exercise before and will again, and tell you that you don't have the time. You simply have to shut these voices down. You know that what you are doing is the very best thing you possibly could be dong to benefit yourself. Nothing else matters. Just do it!

Tactic #12: Exercise Early in the Morning. Training first thing in the morning is a very smart move. It allows you to get your workout in before the demands of your day threaten to overload you. You are also far more focused and energized in the morning. Plus, a good workout will get your day off to a terrific start.

Tactic #13: Recruit Family Support: It is very difficult to maintain regularity of exercise if your spouse or your kids resent the fact that you are doing so. The key to getting them on board is communication. Let your spouse know how important it is to you that you meet your daily exercise goal.

Make it clear how a healthier, fitter you will benefit the entire family. The same goes with the kids. Tell them that you want to be able to remain fit and active in order to do things with them as you grow older. Exercise with your kids as much as you possibly can.

Tactic #14: Block Out your Workout Time: Schedule your exercise sessions into your daily planner as non-negotiable 'you' time. Make it your priority.

Tactic #15: Find a Substitute Activity. There will be times when you simply cannot do your scheduled workout. Maybe the car has broken down and you can't get to the gym. That doesn't mean that you can't do any exercise. Nothing will stop you from doing a bodyweight circuit training program right in your own backyard. If it's raining, do it in your living room. But don't allow the fact that your first option is no longer on the table, men that you do nothing at all.

Keep moving.

Chapter 6: Conclusion

Congratulations.

You have now negotiated your way through the basics of exercise for weight loss, muscle tone and vibrant health. You've learnt exactly what it takes to develop and maintain a fitness lifestyle. Whether working out at home or in the gym, you've been provided with the blueprint to bring it with the very latest in equipment and fat scorching workout programs that will get you to your goals faster than anything else out there.

You've also been equipped with a full arsenal of mental strategies to enable you to overcome procrastination, nix negative thinking and transform your mind into an unstoppable goal seeking force of willpower.

You now have the knowledge.

The question facing you now is . . .
What are you going to do with all of this knowledge?

Are you going to unleash it's power, allowing it to forge your fitness future . . .

OR

Are you going to slink back to the couch, grab another packet of Oreos and dismiss the whole fitness thing as temporary bout of delusion.

You have the power to do either.

Your body is betting on you to make the right choice.

And so are we.

Exercise Glossary

A

Alternating Dumbbell Curl

Stand with dumbbells at your sides, palms turned in toward your thighs. Set your feet shoulder width apart.

Keeping your elbows in at your side, rotate your right wrist and curl that dumbbell to your shoulder. Contract the bicep tightly. As you return to the start position, rotate the left wrist and curl it up to shoulder level. That is one rep. Continue alternating arms to complete the required number of reps.

B

Barbell Curl

Stand with a barbell in your hands, holding it with a shoulder width, underhand. Angle your palms inward. Allow the bar to hang at arm's length in front of your waist. Pull your shoulders down and back and hold them that way. Imagine that you're trying to create as much space between your ears and shoulder as possible. Your feet should be shoulder width apart.

Keeping your upper arms stationary, curl the bar up to your shoulder level. Contract the biceps tightly and then slowly lower the weight to the start position. Completely straighten your arms in the bottom position.

Do not swing your back throughout this exercise – the only movement should be through the forearms.

Barbell Hack Squat

Hold a barbell at arm's length behind you back, with an overhand grip. Your feet should be shoulder width apart. Look up throughout the movement. Maintaining a neutral spine, lower your body down into a full squat. When your hamstrings are parallel to the floor, rise back to the start position.

Bench Press

Lie on a bench and grasp a barbell with an overhand grip a little wider than shoulder width. Hold the bar above your sternum at arms length.

Bring the bar directly down until it lightly touches your torso. Then, keeping your elbows in at your sides, push the bar back up to the starting position, concentrating on contracting the chest. Bring your shoulder blades together as you do the movement.

Bent Over Barbell Row

Stand, holding a barbell with an overhand grip, at a little wider than shoulder width. Hold the bar at arm's length. Bending at the knees and hips, lower your torso until it is at a 45-degree angle to the floor. Maintain a neutral spine and allow the bar to hang straight down from your shoulders.
Pull the bar up to your rib cage, by raising the elbows and squeezing the shoulder blades together. Slowly lower to the start position.

Box Jump

Stand in front of a box or bench, that comes up to your mid thigh. Your feet should be shoulder width apart. Now jump with both feet together to put yourself on top of the bench or box. Now return to the start position. Continue this up and down movement to complete your reps or allocated time, going as fast as possible.

C

Close Grip Bench Press

Lie on a bench and hold a bar above your chest at full arm's length. Your hands should be close together, with thumbs almost touching. Lower the bar to your sternum and then push through the triceps to return to the stat position.

D

Deadlift

Load a barbell and stand in front of it so that it rests against your shins. Bend at the hips to grab the bar with an overhand grip, placing your hands just beyond shoulder width. Keep your lower back slightly arched, in the neutral position. Straighten your arms.
Maintaining a neutral spine, pull the torso back up, thrusting your hips forward and rising with the barbell.

Keep the bar close to your body as you come up.
Lower and repeat for the required number of reps.

Dumbbell Deadlift

Place a pair of dumbbells on the floor in front of you. Bend at your knees to grab the dumbbells with an overhand grip. Straighten your arms and maintain a slight arch in your lower back. Keep the chest up.

Maintaining a neutral spine, rise up to a standing position. As you come up, pull your torso back and up, simultaneously thrusting your hips forward. Return to the start position and repeat for the required number of reps.

F

Fitness Ball Wheelbarrow

Kneel down with a Fitness ball in front of your thighs. Keep your spine in a neutral position and pull your navel in towards your spine. Relax your

shoulders and place your hands on the ball.
Lean forward over the ball until your hands touch the floor and the ball supports your body weight. Feel how pushing onto your hands supports your weight. Push out over the ball, walking your hands out so that the ball is underneath your thighs. Keep your navel pulled in towards your spine to help keep your hips and lower back straight. Walk your hands back in towards the ball.

J

Jumping Split Squats

Standing, feet together, and with hands on hips, bend your knees and jump up, landing with your right foot in front of you and your left foot behind. You'll want to get as deep a bend in your knees as possible. Move immediately into a jump squat in the other leg. Repeat for the required number of reps without pausing.

L

Lunges

Hold a pair of dumbbells by your sides and stand with feet shoulder width apart. Maintaining a tight core, take a big step forward on your right leg and lower your body so that the left knee almost touches the ground. Pause and then push back to the starting position.

M

Mason Crunch

Sit with your back arched and knees slightly bent. Your feet should be just off the floor. Now grasp your hands together in front of your knees. Use a twisting motion to touch your hands to the floor on either side of you in a fast paced motion. Be sure to make solid contact on each side and keep your feet up throughout. Both sides counts as one rep.

Modified Pull Ups

Set up a horizontal bar at hip height. Position yourself underneath the bar and grab it with a slightly wider than shoulder-width overhand grip. Hang from the bar so that your arms are straight.

Squeeze the shoulder blades together as you pull your chest up towards the bar. Keep your body straight and rigid throughout the movement.

Military Press

Hold a barbell in an overhand grip while standing with feet shoulder width apart. Hold the bar at shoulder level so that it runs across your clavicle. Keep your core tight and maintain a neutral spine.

Push the bar straight overhead, without using body momentum. The force should come from the deltoids. Slowly lower and repeat.

P

Pull Ups

Grasp a pull up bar with an overhand grip that is slightly wider than shoulder width apart. Hang completely at arm's length. This is the position you must return to at the completion of each repetition. Cross your ankles over one another.

Pull you chest up to the bar by bending the elbows and pulling your upper arms down while squeezing your shoulder blades together. Come up until the top of your chest just touches the bar. Now, lower your body back to the start position.

R

Resistance Band Overhead Triceps Extension

Adjust your suspension trainer to mid-length.
Standing facing away from the suspension trainer anchor point, with your feet about three feet in front of it. Grab the suspension trainer handles in an overhand grip and extend your arms out straight so that they are in line with your forehead.

Stretch out the straps by leaning into the handles.
Keeping your elbows in (imagine that there is a basketball between them),

lower your forehead down to meet the handles.

Use the power of your triceps to push back to the start position.

S
Seated Cable Row

Sit in front of a low pulley machine with your knees slightly bent and feet braced. Grab the bar with an overhand grip. Sit up right with a neutral spine and your chest up.

Pull the bar to your rib cage. Do not move the position of your upper body throughout the movement. Rather, feel the power of the pull coming from your latissimus muscles in the upper back. Slowly lower and return.

Squats (Body Weight)

Stand with your feet shoulder width apart. Maintain a slight arch in your lower back. Keep your core tight. Stretch both arms out in front of you at shoulder level. Push your hips back and squat down as far as you can. You should at least go down until your hamstrings are parallel to the floor.

Pause at the bottom position, the push yourself back to the start position. Keep your torso upright and maintain a neutral spine throughout the movement. Keep your weight on your heels rather than your toes as you push up.

Squats (Barbell)

Load a squat rack with a barbell at shoulder level. Enter the rack and un-rack the bar so that it sits across your upper back. Grasp the bar with an overhand grip. Pull your shoulders back to allow the bar to rest comfortably across the shoulder blades.

Feet should be shoulder width apart and you should maintain a neutral spine throughout the movement.

Keeping your torso as upright as possible, lower your body as deeply as you can. You should at least go down until your hamstrings are parallel to the floor. Pause fort a moment in the bottom position and then drive through the heels to rise back up to a standing position.

Suspension Flyes

Adjust your suspension trainer to mid-length.
Facing away from the suspension trainer anchor point, grasp the handles with an overhand grip. Your arms should be slightly bent with your hands together in front of your torso.

Maintaining a neutral spine and a tight core, lean into the movement, with your feet together and about 18 inches back from your hands.

Move the arms out to the side until they are at the line of your shoulders. Keep them slightly bent throughout the movement.
Feel the contraction in the chest and then slowly, and with control, return to the start position.

Suspension Knee Tucks

Adjust your suspension trainer to three quarter length.
Position yourself on the floor facing away from the suspension trainer anchor point.
Resting on your elbows, loop your feet into the suspension handles.

Straighten out your body into a suspended plank position.
Maintaining a neutral spine, draw your feet up towards your elbows. Your glutes should rise into the air during the movement.
Slowly straighten the legs back to the start position.

Suspended Plank

Adjust your suspension trainer to three quarter length.
Position yourself on the floor facing away from the suspension trainer anchor point.

Resting on your elbows, loop your feet into the suspension handles. Straighten out your body so that it is in a suspended plank position. Your only contact with the floor should be your elbows. Maintain a neutral spine and a tight core.
Tuck in your pelvis by squeezing your glutes. Now hold this plank position for 20 seconds. Try to increase your time by 5 seconds every workout.

Suspension Push Ups

Adjust your suspension trainer to mid-length.
Face away from the suspension trainer anchor point, grabbing the handles in an overhand grip. Bring your hands together. Keeping a neutral spine (a straight line from the tailbone to the top of the head) and your core tight, lean into the movement, with your feet together and about 18 inches back from your hands.

Bring your torso towards the floor as your hands spread apart. Come as deep into the movement as you can to feel a deep stretch in the pectorals.
Keep the core extremely tight as you slowly return to the start position.
To make the exercise more difficult, move your feet back further toward the anchor point.

Suspension Single Leg Romanian Deadlift

Adjust you suspension trainer to mid-length.

Stand in front of the suspension trainer facing towards the anchor point. Grasp the handles iwithan overhand grip.

With feet shoulder width apart, lower the torso to the front as you push the trainer handles down in an arc. At the same time kick one leg out behind you , ensuring that the leg remains straight. Go slowly and feel for the stretch in your glutes and hamstrings as you raise your leg as high as possible.

Return to start position.

Suspension T-Pull

Adjust your suspension trainer to mid-length.
Stand facing the anchor point and grab the handles in an overhand grip. Lean back so that your body is on a 30-degree angle with the arms extended and handles together.

Pull the handles apart to bring your body to an upright position. Make sure that your arms are locked and the movement is being initiated through the upper back.

Hold the peak contraction for a second and then lower very slowly back to a 30-degree position.

Suspension Triceps Extension

Adjust your suspension trainer to mid-length.
Stand facing the anchor point and grab the handles in an underhand grip. Bend your elbows so that your arms form a right angle at your sides.
Keeping the elbows locked in at your sides, lean back to stretch out the straps.
Perform a triceps extension by pushing your arm down to full extension.
Forcefully contract the triceps in the bottom position before slowly returning to the start position.

Suspension Swimmer Pull

Adjust the suspension trainer to mid-length.
Stand facing the anchor point and grab the handles in an overhand grip.
Push the handles to fully extend your arms at your sides, with the palms facing down.

Take a step back, placing your left foot
behind your right foot.
Keeping your body in a line lower down
into a plank position, where your body is
at about a 20-degree angle. Your front
foot should come of the floor slightly.
Keeping your shoulders down, drive
back up through the lats, to return to the
start position.